Encouragement for when you are told...

YOU HAVE CANCER

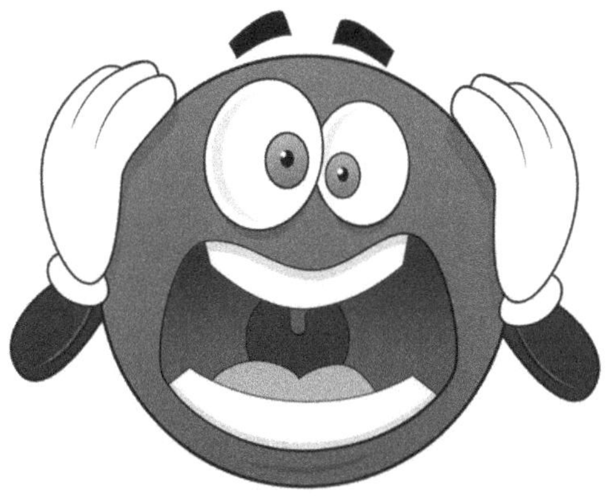

Robert C. Paxton II
and Rebecca Khune

Illustrated By Chad Thompson

Illustrated by Chad Thompson

Printed in the United States of America

Second Printing, 2024

ISBN 979-8-89390-024-8

Library of Congress Control Number: Pending

Ordering Information: Special discounts are available on quantity purchases by bookstores, corporations, associations, and others. For details, contact the publisher at sales@braughlerbooks.com or at 937-58-BOOKS.

For questions or comments about this book, please write to info@braughlerbooks.com

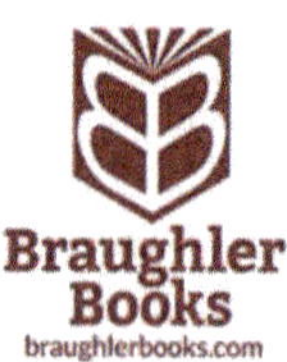

DISCLAIMER

This book presents the research and ideas of its authors.

It is an educational guide that provides general health information with no warranties of any kind, expressed or implied.

The information contained within is not intended to provide specific physical or mental health advice.

The contents of this book should not be construed as medical advice, professional diagnosis, or specific treatment to any individual. It is not a substitute for professional medical diagnosis and care.

Never disregard professional medical advice or delay seeking treatment due to the information contained herein.

The book proper is also
being marketed under the title:
CANCER WHEN THE BAR IS SET HIGH.

To all like me,
called to navigate
through the storm
that is Cancer.

May you gather
inspiration and
support from me, as
I have from others.

- Robert C. Paxton II

It needs said this booklet would never have been written without Rebecca. It was she who suggested doing it and offered her help.

Rebecca wrote the majority of it, in addition to taking my script and bringing my thoughts to life.

She came up with the idea of the accompanying pictures, in each section, in her effort to insert a little levity into a very serious subject.

She found, contracted with, and coordinated with, a remarkable illustrator, possessing notable credentials, who easily portrayed her concepts.

Her desire to inspire people to embrace health and not settle for the mediocre, was evident in the researched and diverse material she presented.

Over these past months, Rebecca did almost all of the work as my illness prevented me from helping. As I stated earlier, without her, this, literally, would not have been done and I am grateful for her incredible work ethic.

- Bob

CONTENTS

WHAT HAPPENED TO ME

My name is Robert Paxton. I live in Columbus, Ohio and, thank goodness, only eight minutes from The James Cancer Clinic at The Ohio State University.

I had not been up to par since about 2017. I hadn't put my finger on any specific problem – it just seemed that I had no energy. Maybe it was simply a part of getting older. Maybe not. I didn't allow myself any time to dwell on it as I was a lawyer with a very rigorous schedule. But, I found myself not getting everything done, even with a great paralegal, Mrs. Lisa Pickett, who kept things going for twenty-eight years.

Although, during those two years, I didn't think much about it, I guess – innately – I knew something was wrong with me. They always say, "Your body will tell you if something's not right."

Still, I basically ignored the signs until that day in 2019 when I literally had trouble walking and my son rushed me to a nearby hospital.

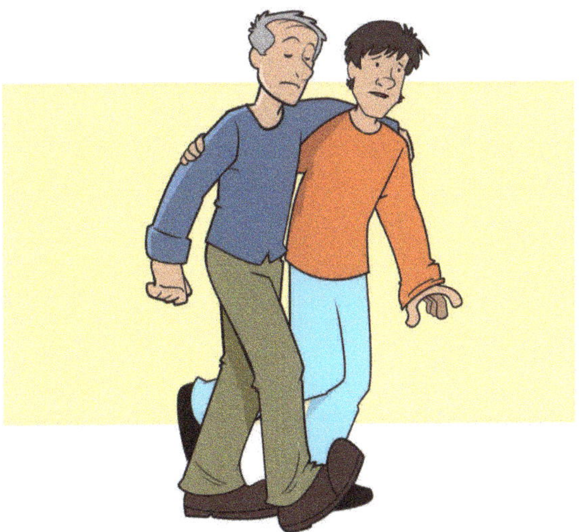

1

There I would
stay for a ten-day
confinement, a
captive of
my bed, since I
was classified as a
"fall risk".

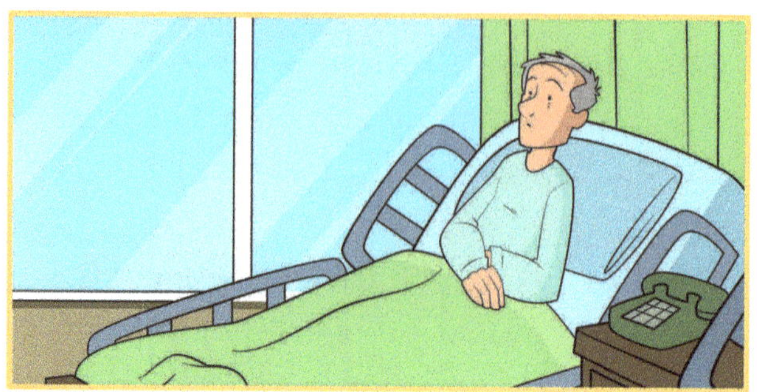

This was a wake-up call where I could no longer occasionally think something might be wrong. I now knew I had a problem. Even though this hospital stay was the beginning of a steady down-hill slide, it would be two more years, in 2021, before the doctors figured out what was wrong.

During this ten-day stay, an unbelievable thing happened. I was told by a staff physician that I had suffered a PULMONARY EMBOLISM – which is a blockage to a lung. I was placed on a blood thinner, observed, and discharged.

On one of my many trips back to the hospital, I inquired as to how this embolism could have happened.

The doctor treating me was someone I had encountered in my many years in law practice. He reminded me that I had been admitted as a "fall risk", so I was not allowed to be up and moving about. No exercise.

He told me, "You can't lay in a hospital bed for ten days and not expect this to happen." I was astonished at his response.

2

Over the next two years, still not feeling well – with no energy – I continued to seek medical help. On one of my now-routine-visits to the hospital, my world shattered. It was forever changed.

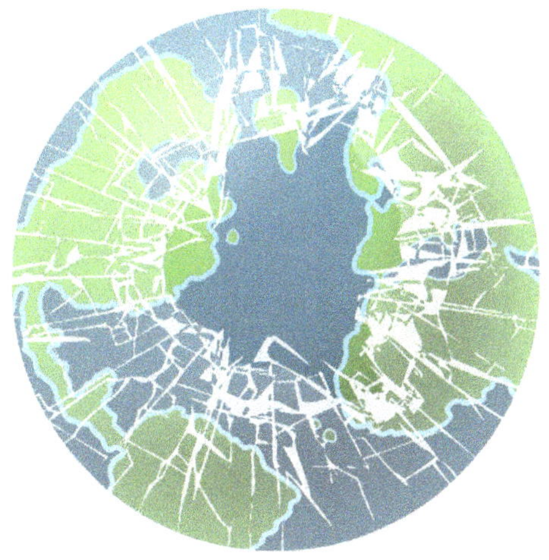

I was not in the least prepared for what came next. My designated doctor came into my hospital room and, as I remember it, stated to me, "By the way, Mr. Paxton, you have cancer."

She left as fast as she had entered.

I was stunned.

Now what do I do?

It took a minute.

The wind had not just been LET out of my sails – it had been violently sucked out!

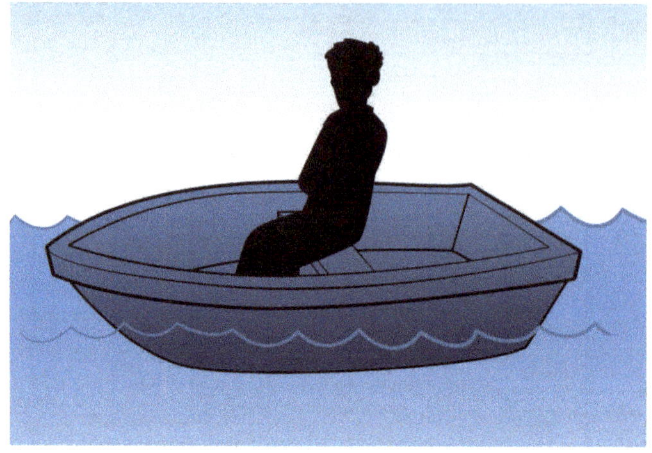

I certainly felt dead in the water.

This point in time, as difficult as it is, requires your best critical thinking. As a friend now tells me, there is more than one avenue of healing to try. Allopathic. Functional. Integrative. Traditional. Eastern medicine. Cleansing, fasts, and foods. Energy medicine. Oxygen and ozone. Light therapy. Combinations of more than one therapy.

Some are therapies on their own, even so, most can also be used as adjunct treatment.

This is all new to me and it's a lot to have to think about. If you are interested in other options, now might be a good time to research if you haven't done so already.

For me, the allopathic treatments of surgery, radiation, and/or chemotherapy were the only ones I was aware of, so I was searching for the best hospital to seek that type of care.

4

Not being a man of inaction, I spent some time speaking with my family and many of my trusted friends, seeking their opinions, life experiences on the matter, and advice.

I immediately changed my care and treatment to The Ohio State University, James Cancer Clinic.

My story moved on from there, as literally, a new chapter began.

Of course, like anyone, I felt that, "This is it – I'm going to die."

But I was a perfect patient. Quite naturally, since I had chosen this clinic, I did everything that The James told me to do.

I had wonderful family support and I would always go to The James with either my son or my daughter.

Routinely, I would be taken to an infusion room, where I would spend four hours being injected with chemotherapy.

For the first time though – as a newbie to chemo – this was quite an experience. While I must say that everyone at Ohio State was very caring and meaningful in what they were doing for me, here's WHAT THEY DIDN'T TELL ME!!!

THE BATTLE WITH CONSTIPATION

What can chemotherapy do to you?

I found out the hard way (no pun intended).

At the first of many infusion sessions, it is part of the nursing staff's job to inform the patient that there can be adverse effects to chemotherapy.

Like:

• Loss of hair;

• Loss of weight;

• Loss of all energy (something I already had too little of); and,

• Unexpected bouts of vomiting.

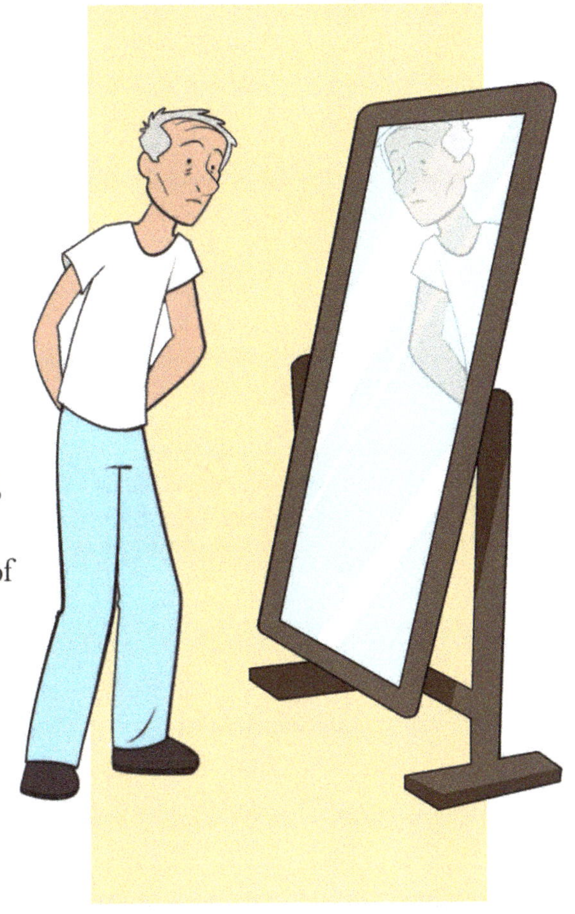

We've all heard this list – frequently. However, with my first round, none of these things happened to me!

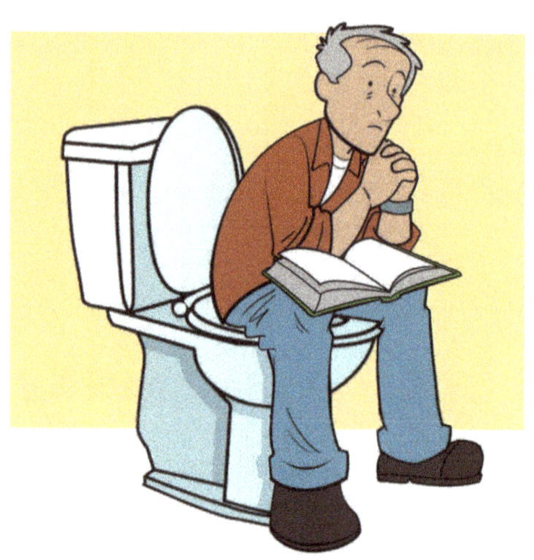

What did happen is this. I became extremely constipated and knew something was wrong. Unable to bear it any longer, finally, on the Friday after the first chemo session at the James, I was admitted again for THREE DAYS in an extensive regiment to get me "unconstipated." I left the hospital on Sunday.

I had never been warned about this possibility. The hospital staff had never made me aware that this condition was "more likely than not" to be an after-effect of a chemotherapy treatment.

So, for any "first-timers" out there, ready to undergo chemotherapy, please accept my WARNING!!! Do something prior to treatment to facilitate ease of movement, and/or have something ready to deal with the problem should it happen to you. It could save you a lot of discomfort and money. Hospital stays are NOT cheap.

Wise advice is, "You have say over your own body. You are in control of what anyone, medically trained, or not, can do to your body." This is, of course, true. But, it took me a long time to realize this basic principle.

So, what was the first thing I did when I got to The James Cancer Clinic on Chemotherapy Day? Of course, I was directed to the infusion preparation room where a nurse put an IV in my arm for the upcoming procedure of a four-hour infusion of chemotherapy.

Nobody Like Needles

My tactic was to look away from the whole process and pinch the inner thigh of my right leg. I thought that I could make myself hurt worse by my self-infliction of pain, than the pain from the needle itself. I tried to distract myself.

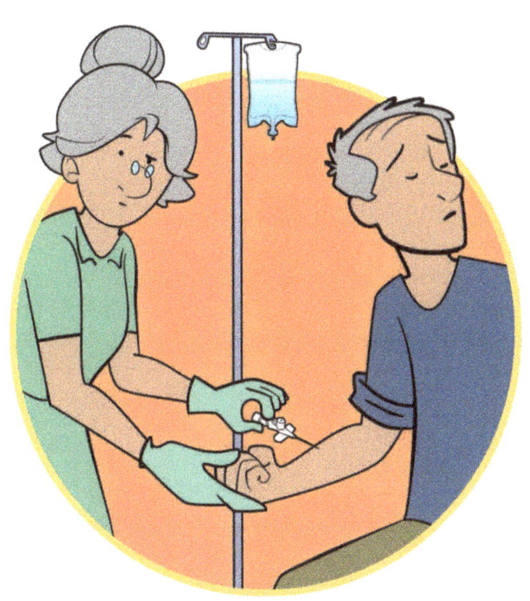

That rarely worked.

One day, in the
preparation room, a
young nurse pricked
me five (5!) times and
still could NOT find a
good vein.

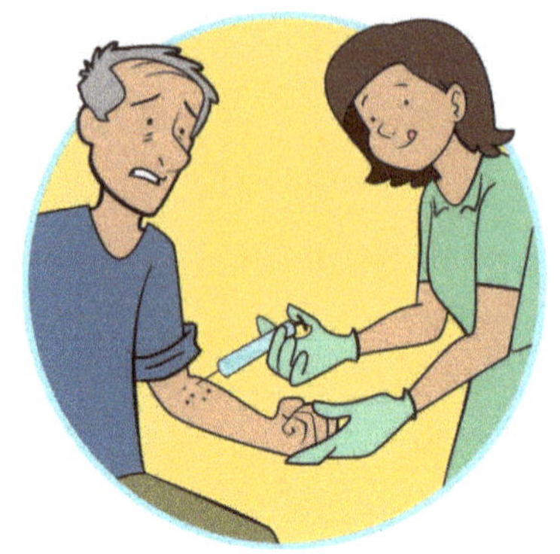

Out of the blue came an elderly nurse, who took charge, and
said, "I can handle this." My arm and I were both hoping like crazy
that she could!

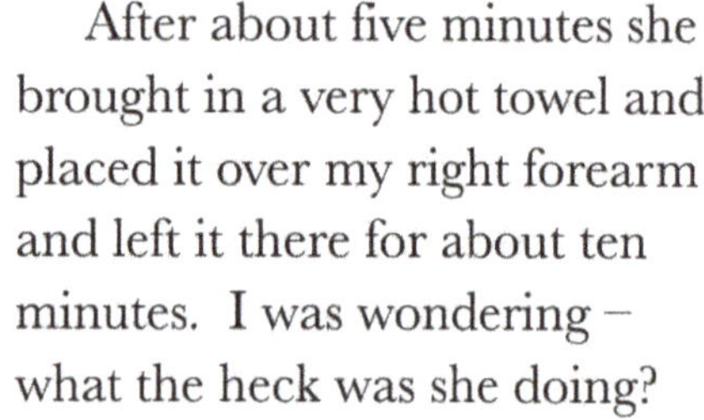

After about five minutes she
brought in a very hot towel and
placed it over my right forearm
and left it there for about ten
minutes. I was wondering –
what the heck was she doing?

She knew.

The hot towel raised ALL
my veins in my forearm.

The needle was inserted, I
felt absolutely nothing, and this
trauma was finally ended!

You DO have say over your own body. Before ANYONE
tries to find a vein in your arm, tell them that you want the
"good ole Mr. Paxton treatment", you want a hot towel
IMMEDIATELY. It is a lifesaver.

It's now 2023 and I have a follow-up note that shows how
much one does have to be their own advocate. Remember, you
are representing you. You are paying people to treat you.
Basically, you have hired them. They work for you. You pay for
their knowledge and advice, but you get to make the decisions.

On my last visit to the infusion room, I was assigned an older,
more experienced nurse. I told her about the towel (as I always
do now) that I needed to do the needle process and – guess
what? She had a plastic-like, or rubber-like, bottle that she
cracked – which immediately got hot – and placed on my
forearm! The usual hot towel was also wrapped around my
arm, which kept the bag in place and added a second source of
heat. She left this on about five minutes.

This made it very clear to me that it's not that these nurses
do not know this trick, they just apparently never tell the patient.
It's up to us to find our voice. Speak up and insist on it!

WHAT – BESIDES CHEMO- IS IN THAT PLASTIC BAG THAT HANGS OVER YOUR BODY DURING THE FOUR-HOUR INFUSION PROCESS? STEROIDS!!!

When I would get home from a chemotherapy treatment, I always had so much energy. This was mind-boggling! I had not had good energy for about four years prior to the cancer diagnosis.

With the steroids, I was usually awake all night, and even spent ONE NIGHT writing a book draft. I had always wanted to put down in writing all of my experiences as a lawyer after fifty years in the practice. I got a lot done in just that one night. I was super-charged.

So, what was making me feel this way? I was later told that the chemotherapy bag contained steroids.

No wonder I felt like I could walk through a glass window!!

So, if you feel this way, it's quite likely steroids and you can talk with your doctor about what steroids can do for you, and what they do to you.

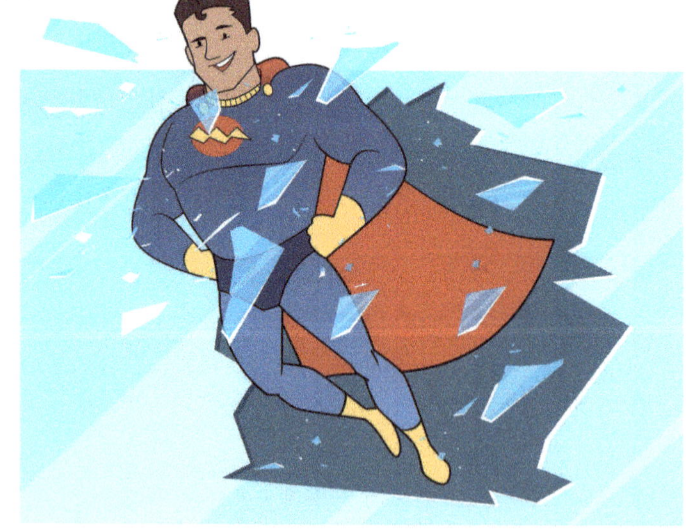

During this past year, to help address my fatigue and poor energy issues, I have taken a few different herbal supplements, recommended by a friend, which I feel have assisted me. I also used plant supplements and melatonin to get me through a time when I had trouble sleeping.

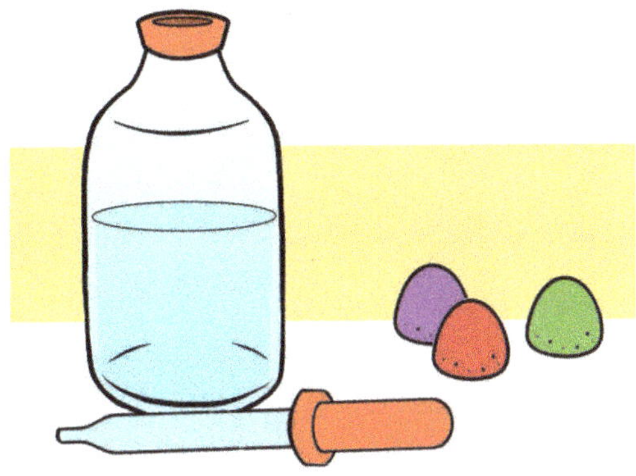

I would say, don't be afraid to reach into other bags of healing to help you on this journey. It's a hard one to navigate.

Keep in mind that people don't all respond the same to either chemical preparations or to herbal remedies. Be mindful of combinations and consult with your doctor.

Be sure to do thorough research about things that are new to you. Perhaps you can find someone who has trusted sources to guide you.

WHAT IS THE RIGHT TEST TO RUN?

I certainly am not a doctor, but I am convinced that I had cancer long before being diagnosed with the same in 2021. For such a long time, I had no energy and was losing my stamina to do little chores, let alone be able to handle a law practice.

At some point in time, it was decided that I should be administered what is known as a **PET** Scan.

The PET (Position Emission Tomography) Scan is an imaging test that checks for diseases in your body. It is an effective way to help discover a variety of conditions, including cancer, heart disease and brain disorders. When used for cancer, providers use it to determine if an area in a patient is cancerous, or to evaluate for any spread of cancer in someone who has already been diagnosed.

The PET-CT, or PET-MRI scanner is a large machine that looks a little like a giant doughnut standing upright – similar to CT or MRI scanners. From start to finish, the procedure takes about two hours to complete.

The special dye, using radioactive tracers, detects diseased cells and can be swallowed, inhaled, or injected into a vein in your arm – depending on what part of the body is being examined. The PET-CT can display multidimensional (3D), color images of the inside workings of the human body. This helps reveal the metabolic or biochemical function of tissues and organs. It can show both typical and atypical metabolic activity – often detecting the atypical metabolism of the tracer in diseases even before the symptoms appear.

In my case, I believe this was the right test for me. Had I known about it, I would have wanted it done sooner. Much sooner.

For you, ask your doctor a LOT of questions about what is right for you. Again, you are your own advocate. Seek other sources if you are not getting clear answers.

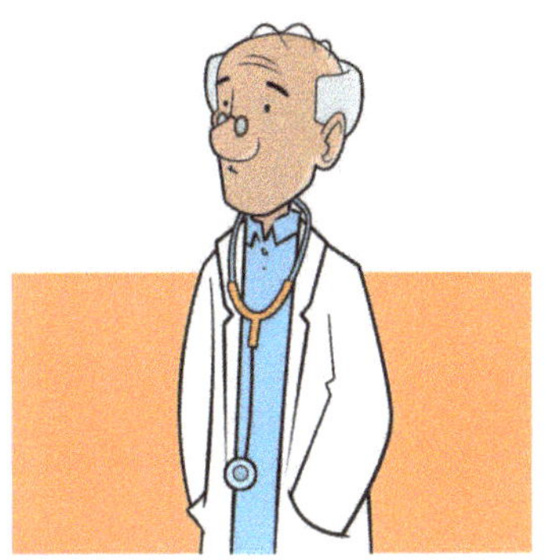

No one doctor knows it all. He only knows as much as his specific training and personal experiences have taught him. He may be a top expert of all those who were taught the same way he was taught, but – and I don't mean to be cryptic – he only knows what he knows. He only was taught what the college he attended chose to teach him.

This is your life, and who you get to treat you is of utmost importance. Choose your doctor wisely.

I believe I was first exposed to the PET Scan at The James, and it clearly showed the many, many lymph nodes in my body. These lymph nodes housed my cancer and were the target for the chemotherapy.

In my case, they do worry about using the PET Scan too much because my kidneys were a little weak going into this. They are holding steady, but it's a good idea not to make them filter too much radioactive dye in their job to process it out of my body.

A second scan, run in 2022, showed no growth.

I can't understand why this test was not run for me earlier. But, as I said, I am not a doctor!!

YOU AND YOUR CELL PHONE
ARE NOW CONJOINED TWINS

I have always, ALWAYS, liked to be current on events in the world. Even while I have been ill, and sometimes homebound, it has STILL been very important for me to stay abreast of what's happening.

I use my cell phone – the handheld computer that it is – all the time. It is a very accessible, portable source of daily going's-on.

That device never leaves my side. Even when I take a shower, it gets put right by the glass door.

5:15 AM. That's what time it was the morning I told myself I wasn't to be satisfied with electronic news – I wanted my newspaper!

It wasn't just very early. It was very dark. Totally dark in fact. The bulb in my porch light had burned out as well as no moonlight.

From my front door there is about six feet of landing and the first six-inch step. Then another six feet, a second step, finally the last landing and last step. THAT was the one that I tripped on a rug, or something, and fell forward.

I landed on my left side, hitting my left shoulder and hip. It really hurt. I know I was a little dazed because, as I laid there, I wasn't quite sure for a bit what had happened. I also wasn't quite sure how long I was there.

I knew the newspaper was between the last step and my car, so I tried to wiggle myself to the car.

I had been pretty weak for a long time, my strength had left me during this illness. Once I was down on the floor, there was no getting myself up. Not without some kind of support.

I'm not sure how long I slid myself along on the walk and pavement, wiggling bit by bit, before I felt the wheel of the car. I followed back to find the driver's door, and then managed to reach up to the handle. I got the door opened with my left hand, and with my right hand grabbing the seat, I was able to pull myself up.

Once seated in my Jeep, I called my son. Apparently he doesn't answer the phone at five in the morning. The second try revealed that neither did my daughter.

I fared better on my third call. "Upper Arlington Police Department."

I'm sure they've heard this many times before. "I fell and I need some help. I made it to my Jeep."

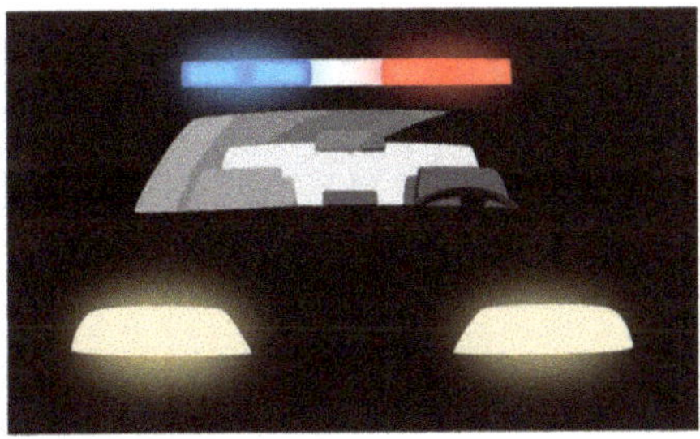

I don't know what the neighbors thought of all of this before six in the morning, with lights flashing AND sirens, but I can tell you, THOSE YOUNG MEN ARE THE NICEST YOUNG MEN IN THE WORLD! That's how you spell C-L-A-S-S.

"What's wrong, sir?"

"I fell."

"What do you want us to do, sir?"

"Just get me in the house."

They were marvelous with how easily they righted me and started helping me to the house door.

As we moved past it, I spied the original object of my morning obsession and, shamelessly, without hesitation, inquired, "Would you pick up my newspaper for me?"

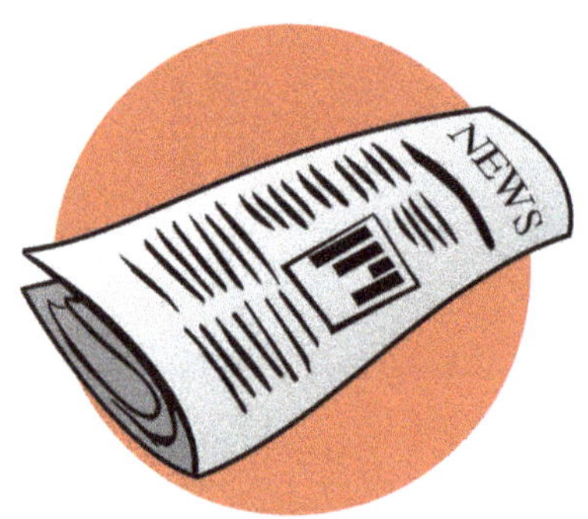

Okay, that was a lot to go through to get a paper delivery, but that's not the point of my telling on myself. NEVER go anywhere, even room to room in your home, when you are weak, frail, or feeble without some sort of a communication device.

If you are trying to live on your own, make sure you have some way to call for help. It really could be a lifesaver.

Does the calf of your leg still yield a firm handful of flesh when you grip it?

Or, does it flop
and wave at you?
Like your arms.

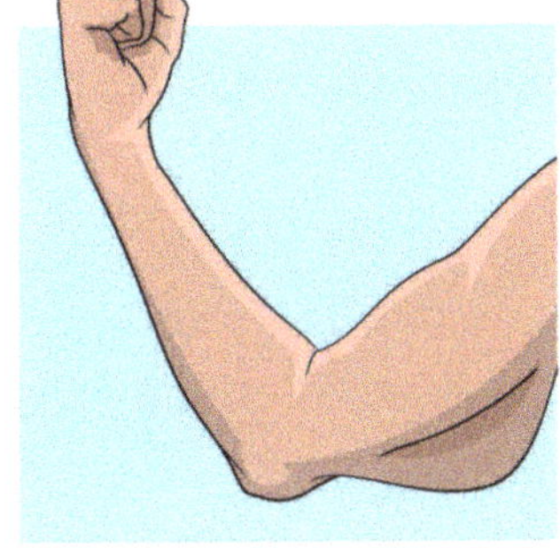

The official definition of this muscle-wasting condition is the degenerative loss of skeletal muscle mass and strength. Most mainstream, conventional, allopathic doctors will further state that it is an unavoidable condition of aging and illness.

This is the frailty that most people take for granted is inevitable. This infirmity is why so many of the elderly and ill fall and sustain injury. This IS the, "I've fallen and can't get up."

No leg strength. No arm strength.

Being an optimistic person who is really beginning to like looking outside-of-the-box, I'm finding there is a lot one can do to greatly slow this down. GREATLY!

I'm checking out about giving my body all the building blocks it needs, then I plan to MOVE it!

I know I have to study what all has to be IN my body for it to even be able to MAKE muscle. It has to have specific ingredients. A lot more than what I'm currently giving it.

Making muscle is serious business. I think it's important to find out what all muscle is made FROM and then make sure the body gets a STEADY supply of it all.

Then, once we have the process of rebuilding the structure in place, we need to strengthen the structure. Work those muscles. A little at a time turns into quite a lot if one keeps at it.

WE MUST BE CONSISTENT. Whether it's a little, or a lot, I think we should keep on a regular schedule – every week. I'm expecting to be amazed at how soon I'll see – and feel – a difference. Even if it's just walking easier. And hopefully not tripping over rugs.

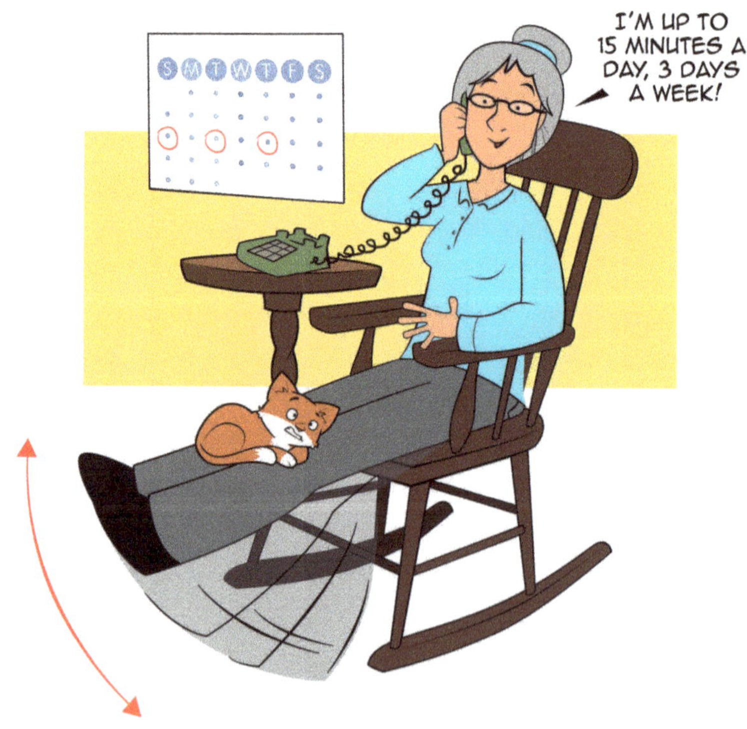

20

To build this muscle, and our bones, resistance exercise is recommended. This is where the body is 'resisting' against a force – for example, a weight. One doesn't need expensive equipment. Use stretch bands and hand weights. We can even use a can of beans in each hand for beginner weights.

As soon as we feel able, we can try 'wall push-ups', or something similar. That's an easy one and it is a 'resistance' exercise. The weight of our own bodies is the 'resistance weight'.

I do want all of us to be strong, but I don't want anyone to overdo it. Please check with your physician to make sure whatever you decide to do is not too much of a strain for you. Depending on how frail you already are, it might be a good idea to have someone with you.

CHECK WITH YOUR DOCTOR AND USE COMMON SENSE.

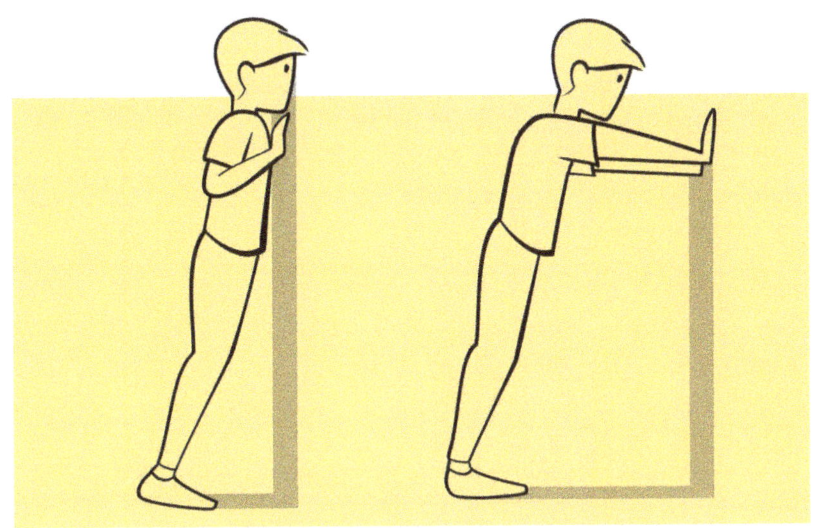

FEET ARE TO BE ONLY AS FAR AWAY
FROM THE WALL AS YOU CAN SAFELY BALANCE.

MY SHOT GLASS IS HALF-FULL
-AND IT'S NOT ALCOHOL

Imagine my surprise one day, while I was eating, when I bit down on something hard. I fished it out and it was a filling. I wasn't prone to losing fillings, so that was unusual.

But, that can happen. I'm sure it happens to someone every day.

But then it happened again when I was eating.

And again.

And it kept happening over the course of the first year after I started the chemo treatments until I had filled the shot glass on my nightstand half way up. I don't think I have any fillings left in my teeth.

These were all the mercury-amalgam fillings that conventional dentists usually place in the chewing teeth. I now have a nice collection of metal.

A web search to see if anyone else had problems with fillings coming out brought up lots of comments about teeth: loosening, falling out, discoloring, and even children whose second set of teeth wouldn't come in.

While my doctors would neither confirm nor deny any correlation, I can only state my experience, and chemo related or not, my fillings did fall out.

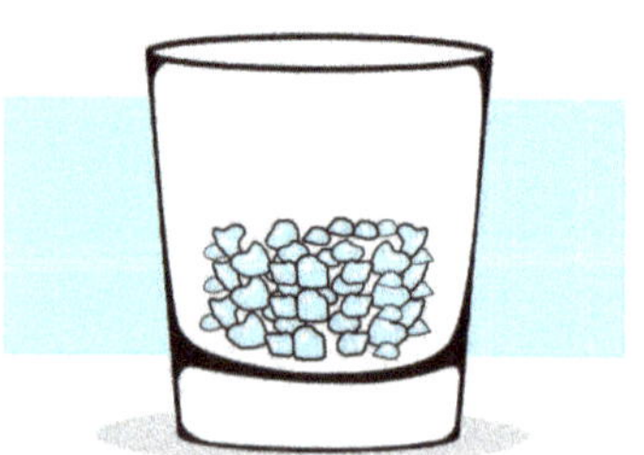

WHY ME? I WAS ALWAYS HEALTHY, WASN'T I?

I completed the six months of chemotherapy the doctor had prescribed for me and have been placed on what The James calls "maintenance treatment".

My diagnosis is a form of cancer known as B-Cell Non-Hodgkin's Lymphoma. As best as I understand it – and I'm still not exactly sure – my cancer is permanent in nature, but treatable.

Even though I am two years into treatment, sometimes the disbelief is still palpable.

How could this have happened to me? It was a low blow. Hard to comprehend. The utter confusion over it all had filled my mind. I didn't understand it. I didn't want to believe it or accept it.

I thought I was healthy. Strong. I was an Eagle Scout.

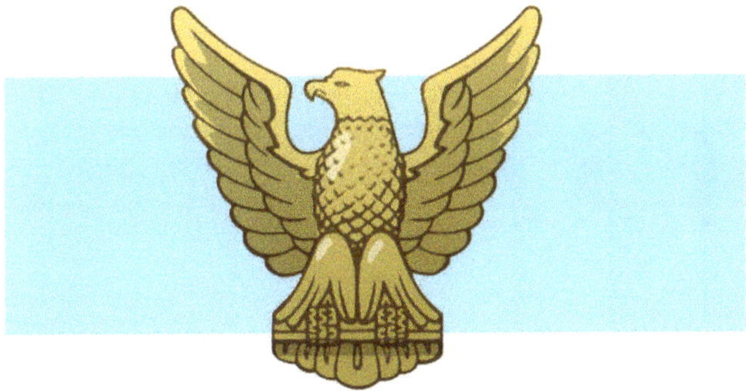

I was an athlete in high school – good enough to earn a scholarship to play college football. I declined the scholarship to that college because I wanted to go to Ohio State.

It was there that I spent seven straight years receiving my law degree, and upon graduation carried on that profession for over fifty years.

While there, I was proud to have been an Ohio State Letterman for the OSU Track Team.

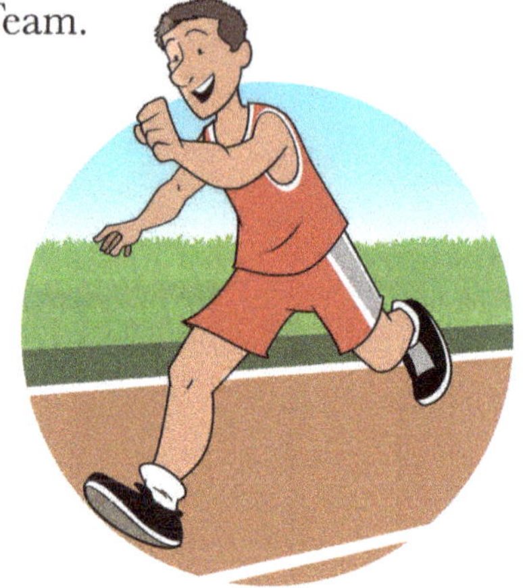

Carrying my pole vaulting from high school, I jumped over the bar at fifteen feet. After college, I had refereed pole-vaulting there for a while.

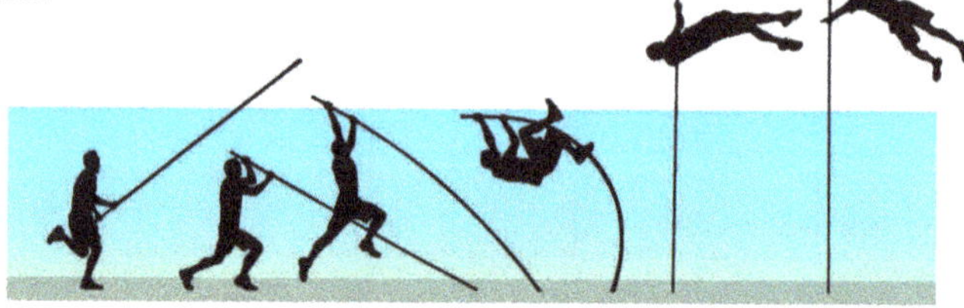

For a bit after that, I ran five miles a day, three times a week.

I was in the army reserves for eight years. My dad had expected me to excel and I strove to do just that.

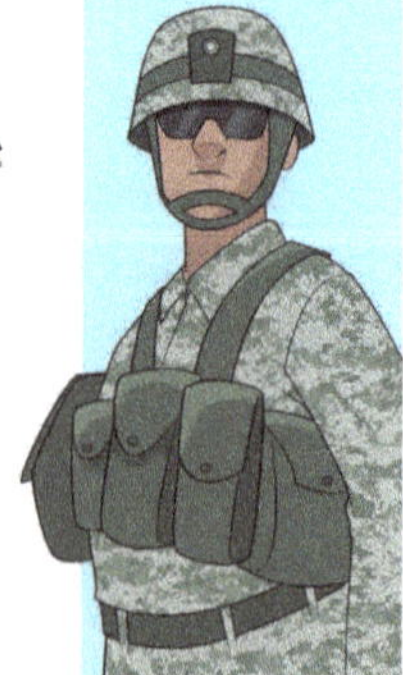

24

Until the diagnosis, I was going through life like everyone else. What did I do wrong? I thought I was doing everything correctly.

The emotions you experience when a doctor says, "You have cancer," are overwhelming. It took everything out of me. It was difficult to wrap my mind around it.

I remember I saw it on TV one time and thought, this could never happen to me.

It didn't matter if one person, or if EVERYONE had felt this way – it was a shock. It's hard. It just didn't compute. It's not something a community can feel – it's personal.

I was blaming myself for messing up, but I hadn't taken into account that exercise and trying to keep one's muscles strong was only one piece of the cancer puzzle.

The assaults to our bodies come from all around us. The chemicals in our food, water, and the air affect us.

As does radiation, EMF's, stress, lack of sleep, loss, depression, emotions (the demons of envy, worry, regret, shame, bitterness, guilt, resentment), plus so many other things that they seem too numerous to count.

Stress and loss are two of the biggest instigators of disease.

If you want to heal (or not get sick in the first place), also remove all of the emotional bogey-men.

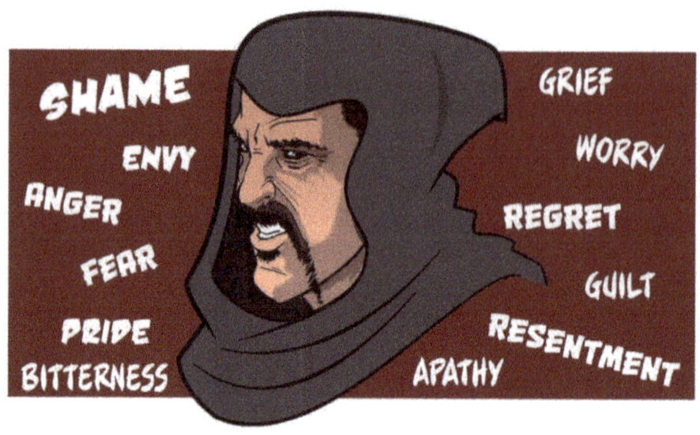

I think sometimes that just the right stuff comes together to construct that horribly threatening, perfect storm.

I bring all of this up because we are called to accept this new fact. Like it or not. CANCER.

We can't go back and 'not get it'. The only direction we can go is forward. But we can be pro-active.

We CAN evict all that "why me" and anger, and replace it with an equal, positive force to try our darnedest to help fight the cancer!

I don't think it can be fought as well with negative feelings present. Deliberately, consciously, replace those with the opposite emotions.

We must try our best to be optimistic and happy. Yes, happy. That's a tall order, but try to grab some good from another part of your life and build on that.

It's hard – really, really hard – for all of us who hear this diagnosis, but my advice to individuals who are going through what I have, and am, is to chew up all of this disbelief and anger.

CHEW IT UP AND SPIT THAT DARK STUFF OUT!

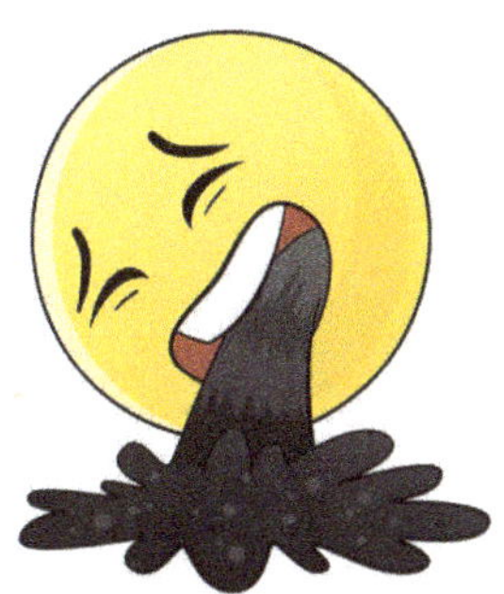

Incredulously, sometimes that "Why me?" becomes "Thank you, God" as we realize that what happened, forced us to dramatically change our lives and become better people. Our soul grew in goodness. As hard as it is, try to see if you can find meaning and purpose in it.

Whatever you feel about that, I hope you can make a plan, have faith, pray a lot, accept help, and dig in for the fight of your life. Try to keep a stiff upper lip, laugh, love, be grateful for what you do have, be generous, help others, and live every day to the fullest.

NUTRITION IS THERAPY

Dinnertime is not something that happens just to get our belly to stop growling.

Our bodies were magnificently designed, intricately so, to run on the fuel of food. The whole process is amazingly complex.

Man can make really efficient machines. BUT, the machines God made (YOU and ME) are even more efficient and can self-heal!

This complex organism must have good fuel to be self-sustained. Just as we would put the best fuel into our vehicles for peak performance, we must do the same with our organic machine.

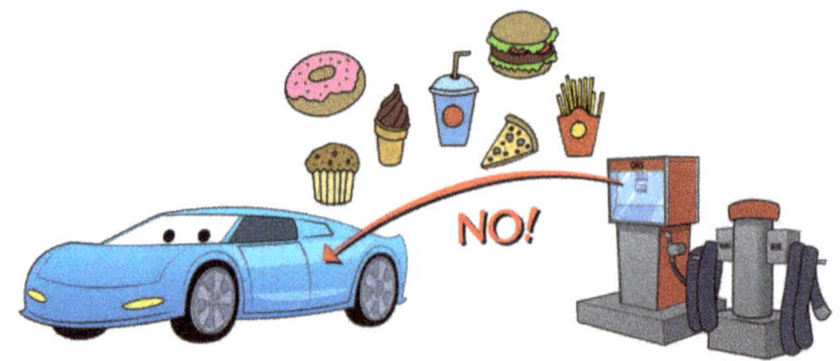

When the race is on, we wouldn't put anything but the best in our cherished car. We need to treat our body at least as well as a car we probably aren't even planning to keep our whole lives.

Our bodies are just sitting there, completely at our mercy, impatiently waiting for us to give them the correct building blocks. Once we have cancer, if we were EVER going to be anal, this would be the time.

What we eat can either keep our body humming, or it can set it up for failure.

28   We know how to pick the right foods.

Let's make it kindergarten-easy. Divide the food into two groups. Things "good" for us; and, things "not good" for us.

There will be occasions where we will not have perfect choices. Just pick the best option available.

We all know we should avoid sugar. Cancer LOVES sugar. Maybe don't give it any.

Are we avoiding processed foods, preservatives, chemicals and dyes? Something to consider.

What if we stopped feeding our indulgences and started feeding our purpose? To get well.

If anyone needs to be convinced how well the body does its job, without us even asking it to, have them observe a cut on their skin just get 'zippered' up and grow over – all on its own.

No doctor waved a magic wand and healed it – it healed itself.

The exact same healing happens internally. Inside of God's work-of-art, tiny repairs are constantly happening to attempt to repair all assaults to the interior of this creation. It does the best job it can, with the tools we have provided. If it's not a perfect fix – then WE probably didn't remove a roadblock that needed taken out (like heavy metals and parasites) and/or, WE didn't furnish enough of the right tools, or even, WE delivered too many inadequate tools along with only a few of the correct ones.

We've made our little 'internal' workers' jobs a lot tougher.

"None of this stuff is on the list of what fuels this process! Who called for these substitutions? Someone has been sending me inferior material for years!"

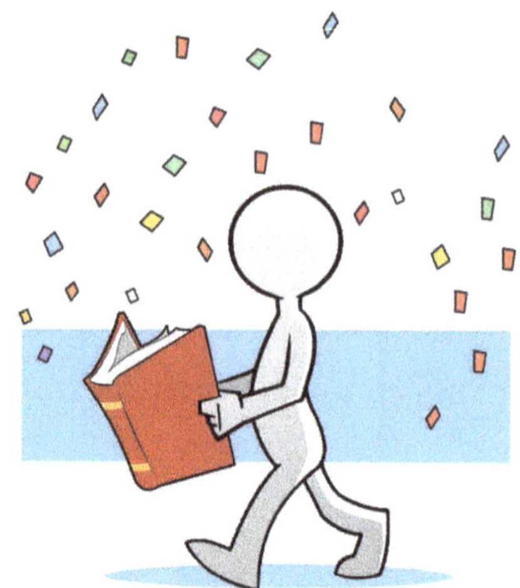

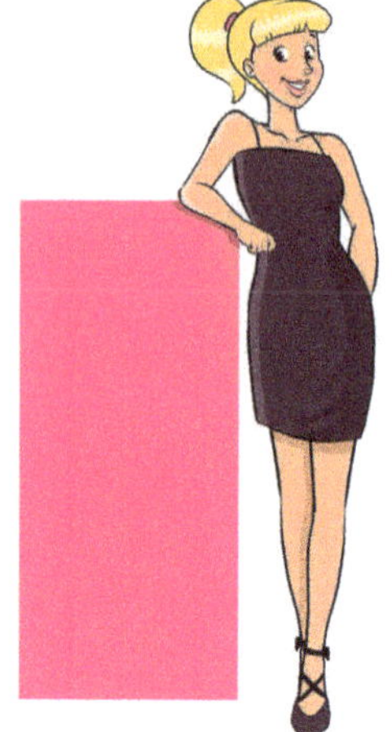

"If you'd just send me the right stuff, this is what God had in mind – okay, maybe that's a little more me than God."

"BUT, this is all I can make with what you've been giving me to work with. I can barely maintain function, yet alone do repairs!"

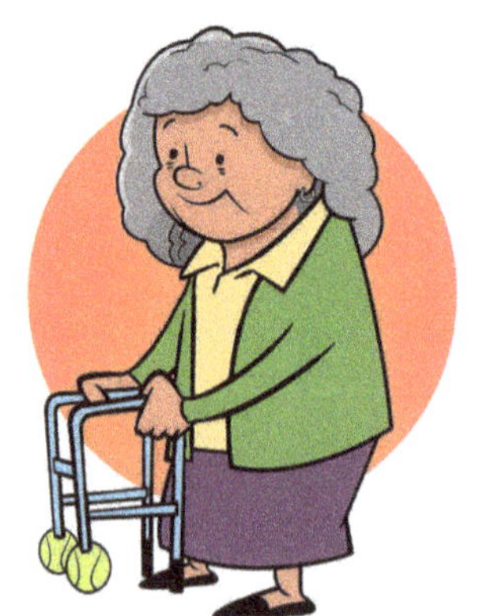

"I don't know how much longer I can keep this equipment going! The parts are starting to malfunction!"

"Tell the boss, we are done if we don't get a major overhaul soon."

Most people have no idea how significant food's role is in healing. Not only is it fuel for energy, it also brings instructions to the cells for regeneration.

You can pretty much tell, just by looking at some people, they are not in good health. Many who look pretty bad on the outside, will be the first to say that they have a lot of medical problems on the inside also.

I'm just thinking that we need to make the effort to become healthier in every way we can, and what we eat is a very important part of all of that.

We have to change our eating habits to help ourselves feel better. Pay attention to Einstein's famous quote about insanity – doing the same thing over and over and expecting different results.

If I may offer a suggestion, I'd consider restoring the gut first. After all, it's not really what you eat, but what you absorb! You want to be making sure all of that good stuff you're putting in actually gets used.

Let's try to eat correctly for a three-month-trial. Then re-evaluate to see if we've improved. The goal is to strengthen the body while the doctor does his thing.

I hope, if we all do our part, that we'll see God's self-healing masterpiece at work.

Let's educate ourselves on this. Become a "foodie". Follow some food gurus online. Watch a digestive health seminar – most are free!

There isn't a lot in life that we can control, but what we eat IS something WE CAN REGULATE!

I think it's a good plan to start doing better today. Please don't wait until you have cancer.

I never saw this coming.

This is such an emotional time in a cancer victim's life, so emotional that you don't really know how sick you are. I certainly did not.

In 2022, my two children revealed to me an awful secret they had been carrying. They had lived with that dreadful burden until I was at least a year past when they had been told.

Imagine their anguish in 2021, when a doctor had told them, "Your father will not make it through Christmas of this year."

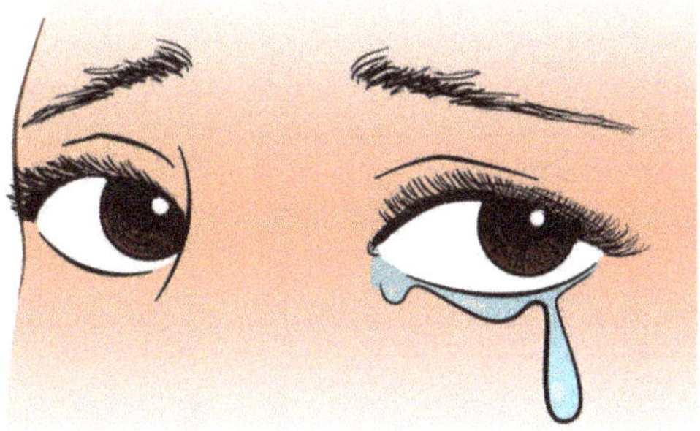

I'm a believer of the truth . . . but, I don't know – would I have given up if I'd been told I'd be dead before Christmas?

I have a fighting spirit, but when your doctor – in whom you have probably put all your trust – pretty much says, "You're gonna die, and I mean SOON!". . . I might have quit.

Granted, the doctor did not give that dire prediction to me, but families are the caregivers and they also need to believe there is some hope.

There is a strong mind/body connection. You – and all around you – simply MUST NOT give in to NEGATIVE thinking. Your body listens to your mind, to your thoughts, even unconscious ones.

There are still a few doctors out there who could glean something from this. In situations like this one,

Brutality is not required. When all optimism is dashed, the prognosis often becomes a self-fulfilling prophecy. The patient – and the family – gives up.

Perhaps the doctor could have said, 'your father has a disease that I don't know how to totally eradicate, however, I have been trained to have treatments administered that can prolong his life for an undetermined amount of time. There are a lot of variables that come into play for how long that will be. There have been patients with this cancer who have not lived long, some have survived for a few years, and there have even been those cases, admittedly not frequently, where a complete remission seems to have happened. We'll do our best and see how it goes. We'll also keep watch for any new advances in this field.' THERE. Truth and Hope. A little humility goes a long way.

Maybe leave out those blanket statements of doom. The doctor had not told me that he believed my shelf life had expired, so I had no clue how sick I was – and for those things I'll be forever thankful!

As of June, 2023, when my latest tests were done, I was given the "green light". I've been told the cancer will come back – maybe next week, maybe in fifty years – but as of now, I'm clear.

I'm still here!!! I celebrate this day!

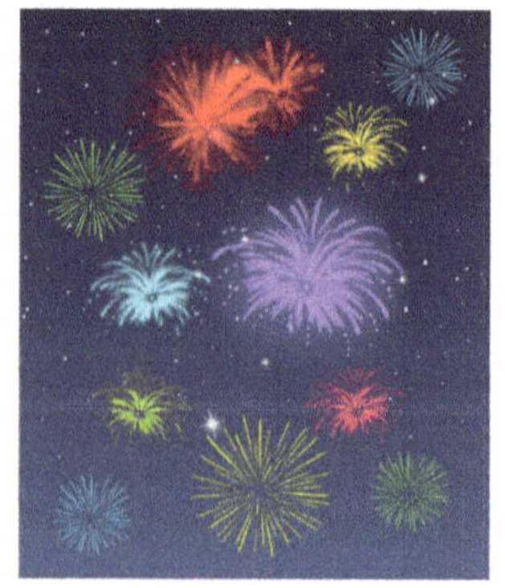

34

Upon leaving the first hospital, my case was transferred to The James Clinic. I had been sent home in a wheelchair and, physically, I was at my lowest point yet.

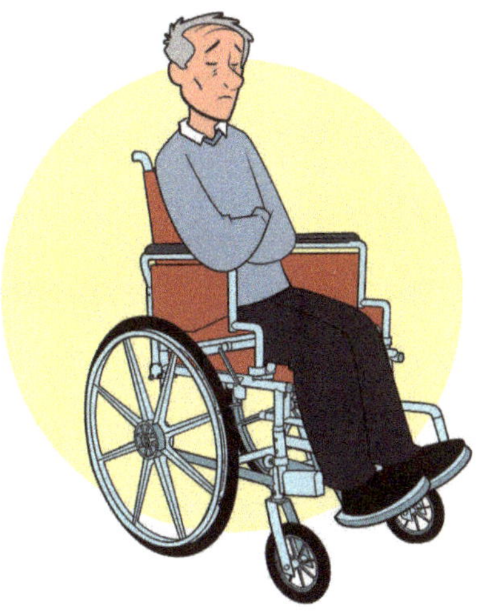

Between being debilitated by long-standing cancer (I still believe it was a late diagnosis) and the pulmonary embolism, I was so weak that I no longer was able to walk.

Despite my obvious troubles, I am a most fortunate man in many ways. My son-in-law has a home health business and provided for me a woman who cared for me 24/7 for thirty days. I was unable to go to the bathroom by myself or to shower. I know so many cancer patients are not able to have the kind of care I received and I am ever-so-grateful for the generosities given to me. I know how much I was given.

I am in my seventies, so Medicare was available to pay for a physical therapy assistant who, at first, came to my home two times a week. His visits tapered off through about a three-month period.

During this time, with the P.T.'s help, I graduated from the wheelchair to a walker. Then from the walker to a cane.

Finally, the physical therapist placed a belt with handles around me (to be able to keep me from falling) and, with his assistance, we would try to walk me continuously around and around the dining room table.

It was a lot of hard work, but the day ultimately came when I said to my therapist (as I played with the famous words of President Ronald Reagan, while in Germany, to the President of Russia, "Mr. Gorbachev, tear down that wall.") "Mr. Therapist, take off that belt." It felt like magic that I was able to walk again all by myself. What a miracle from where I had been!

I think being in ignorance of how sick I was worked in my favor. I didn't know I wasn't expected to get better. I am reminded again of how important it is to keep a fighting spirit. Persistence is key.

Do you remember the movie, Galaxy Quest and the mantra, "Never give up!"?

Words to live by.

After decades of independence, my lack of mobility was really hard to undergo. Everyone had to take care of me and that was a position I was not used to.

I had not driven a car for over two years. What a challenge to overcome!

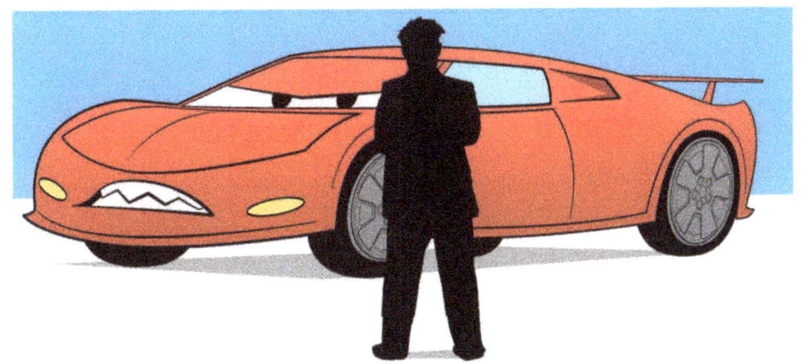

In the summer of 2022, I told myself I had to try doing this.

I was extremely nervous. Having been away from it for so long, all the directional signs and traffic lights made for a very scary optical.

But I kept facing it, and very slowly, I got back into the habit. What a joy to be able to do that for myself. Just to be able to drive to Giant Eagle, my local grocery store, and buy my own groceries!

I take every accomplishment as it comes – no matter how small. I enjoy them while I have them, even if they are not permanent.

This independence lasted only a few months but it was a joy I cherished. Unfortunately, I had taken two steps back and it had again been several months since I've had the pleasure of cruising the streets on my own.

However, now in June of 2023, I was again willing to make a start. I decided to make it out to my car and start it up to run for a bit to keep the battery up. The battery, without my knowing it, had already decided to take a break. Undaunted, I called Triple A.

A very nice gentleman jump-started my car and it was decided that I let it run a bit to 'build up' what I had initially tried to 'keep up'.

It was seven hours later that I remembered the car!

Yes. It HAD run out of gas. And with the ignition key still in the ON position, it had also depleted the battery. Round one – point for the car.

Round two. I again called Triple A. The same, very nice gentleman arrived with gas and jumper cables. THIS TIME I went into the house and set an alarm!

With adequate gas and a charged battery, I squared my shoulders and made for the closest gas station. In for a penny, in for a pound.

I had instant reward for my efforts! While there, I, by wonderful chance, met a former hurdles champion from Ohio State who later went to the Olympics. What are the odds of that! AT A GAS STATION! We had a marvelous conversation. Made my day!

The car may have gotten the first lick in this time, but a successful excursion and fortuitous encounter with a star athlete makes my little jaunt a win/win!

Today I conquered!

Round two – double points to me!

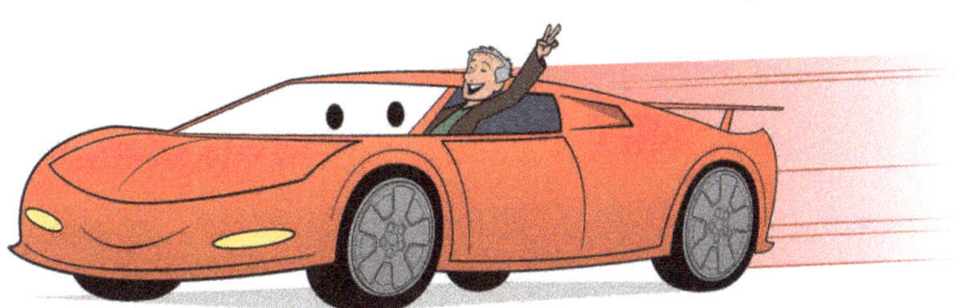

I am very blessed with a GREAT FAMILY. I have two children, twelve grandchildren and five siblings.

I believe I could not have made it through this so-very-trying time in my life without them.

My brothers and sisters would regularly check on me. My grandchildren were also saying, "How's Papa doing?"

But, most importantly, my son and daughter live within a short distance from my home. They have taken me to all of my hundreds of appointments, my chemotherapy treatments, and have supplied me with food and the other essentials I needed to survive. I could NOT have done all of this without them.

They have been, and are, remarkable.

Their love steadies me with every deed done. I feel I can literally bask in its warmth.

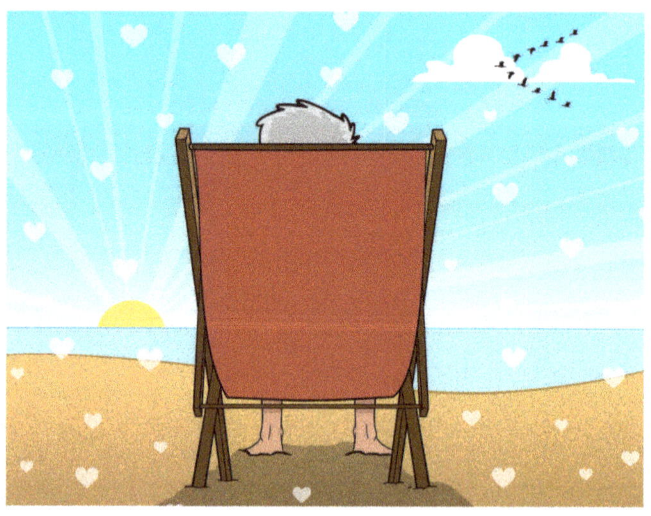

My life has been filled with many good friends, former law buddies, and classmates. They, too, have always been there to help. I remember back to my seventieth birthday when an absolutely fabulous party was set up for me. It's that kind of generosity, almost unexpected – but not really – that I now receive.

Out of my seventy plus years, figures from past and present have stepped up to help. It humbles a person to be the recipient of such compassion.

I feel the same caring from my fellow parishioners at church. A phone call or physical assistance seems to come out of nowhere – and, again, I'm not alone.

If you have family – let them help you. Being the 'giver' has benefits for them also.

I hope if there are rifts in your clan, that you can mend them.

This boils down to support with a capital "S". I obtain it from numerous people. I have been so fortunate in this area. I wish everyone could have this – it's been really important to me.

Maybe you are from a small family, or have few close friends. Even ONE devoted person in your life can fill that role. That would be quality over quantity.

It is healthy for our spirit, our psyche, to have a good hand-holder in our life. It helps to lessen the weight on our own shoulders. Facing a disease like this one is quite a load to carry.

Perhaps, at present, you are all alone and it's all on God. Prayer is your support. Call on Him often. Call on your church. If you don't have one – find one.

It's hard to think of anyone not having lots of comfort in this trying time and I wish that never happened.

Obviously, not everything in my life is a bed of roses, but, it would be perfect if everyone could have this part of my life, because this part is richly blessed.

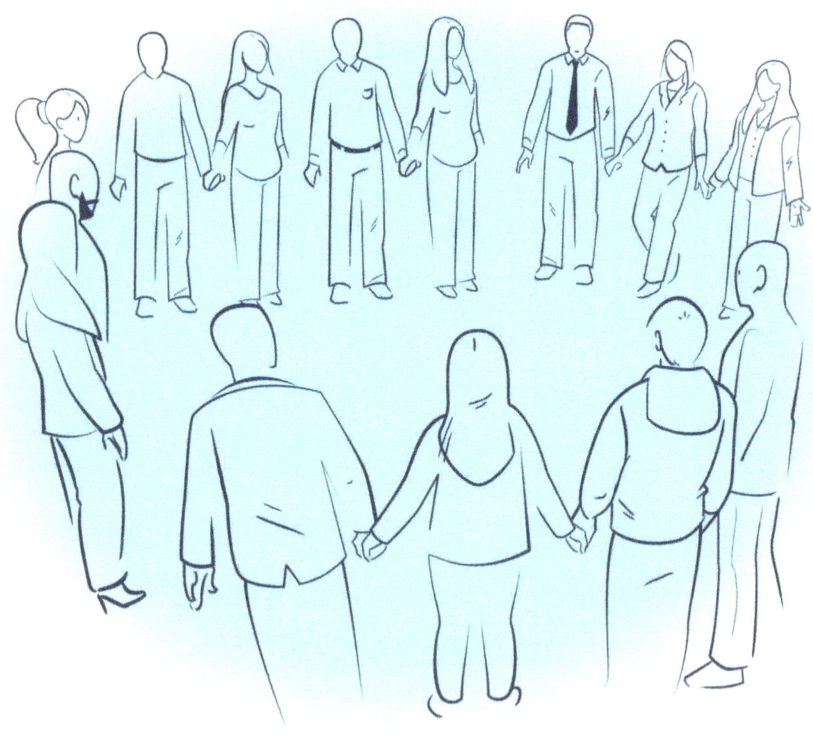

HOW LONG WILL I HAVE
TO BE ON CHEMO?

At an appointment this past year, my daughter asked my doctor, "Just how long does my dad have to be on this chemotherapy?"

He had responded, saying, "Maybe for the next thirty days, the next three years, or for the rest of his life. You have to understand that we're trying to keep your father alive."

WOW! Did that get our attention. As we left the doctor's office to go to the infusion room, I jokingly teased my daughter, "Gosh, we have to take this matter seriously! "

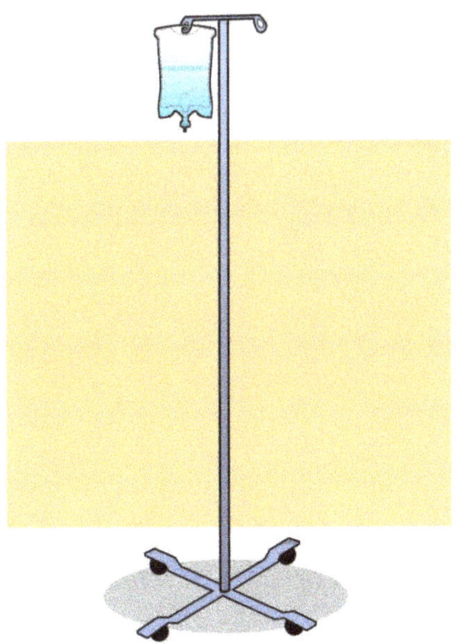

TAG TEAMING WITH YOUR DOCTOR

Any cancer is a battle and I realize that B-Cell Non-Hodgkin's Lymphoma is a tough one to beat.

Communicate with your doctor. Ask him if he is doing anything to help your body heal during the chemo treatments, or is he simply concentrating on killing out and removing cancerous growths?

Is he being the "teacher" (doctor; Latin) and the "healer" (physician; Hebrew), or is he just being the exterminator? Consider the wisdom of Hippocrates.

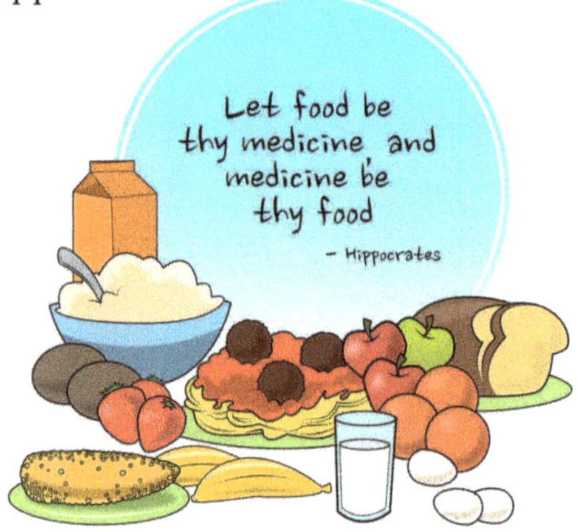

Is your doctor recommending or prescribing anything to help you withstand the damage you sustain from the chemo, or is his vision more of a 'tunnel-vision', looking only at the cancer cells? By compartmentalizing on a single task, he is missing the glorious opportunity to treat the entirety that is YOU!

If he is only concerned with addressing the cancer, then somebody needs to clean up the mess.

That would be YOU. Remember, you are your own advocate.

It is up to you to go the extra mile to find therapies you can be doing, or substances you can be taking, toxins to be removing, and proper foods to be ingesting in order to build up what the chemo has injured.

Look at chemo as a napalm bomb. It is not an intended scorched earth policy approach, but the results can be similar. Your body is not just IN the battlefield, it IS the battlefield.

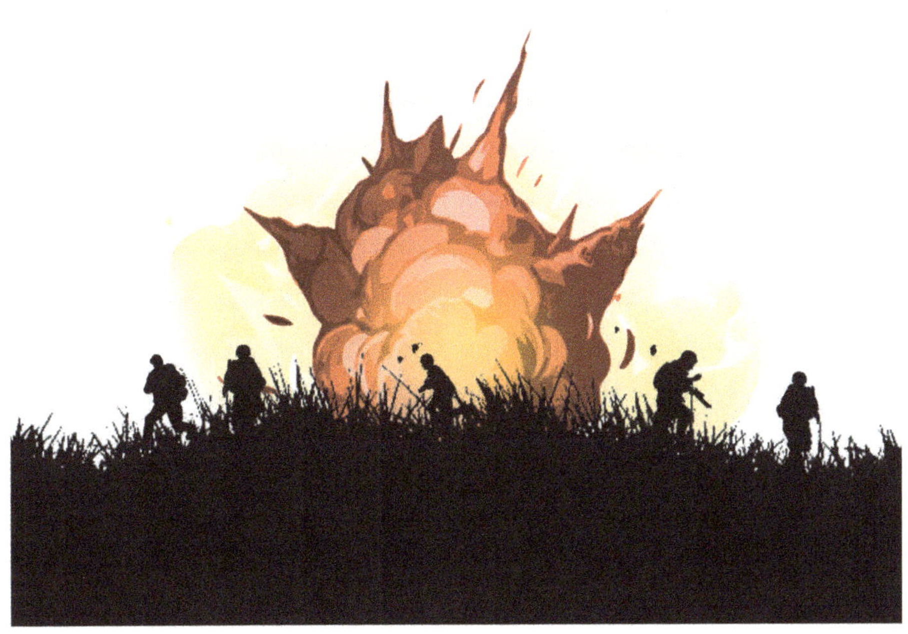

Everything in you sustains collateral damage. Don't be remiss. Deal with that. After all, what could it possibly hurt to try to be healthier!

My understanding of the administration of chemotherapy is that while they are killing out the rogue cells, they hope they don't also kill so many of the good cells to where you can no longer function.

Looking at it that way, one can see how important it is that someone assumes the role of being the strategist to rebuild the battlefield. That war-torn terrain is your brain, your gut, your organs, your blood vessels and everything else from stem to stern.

If you keep taking the hit, time after time, and never rebuild from the damage – ask yourself, "What is the unescapable consequence of that?"

Your chemo doctor is trying to help you survive the cancer. Someone has to help your body survive the chemo. Take this seriously. Don't settle for enduring the chemo – aim to THRIVE!

So, I guess I'm in it for the long haul, and I am still alive! I am still relishing good times with family and friends.

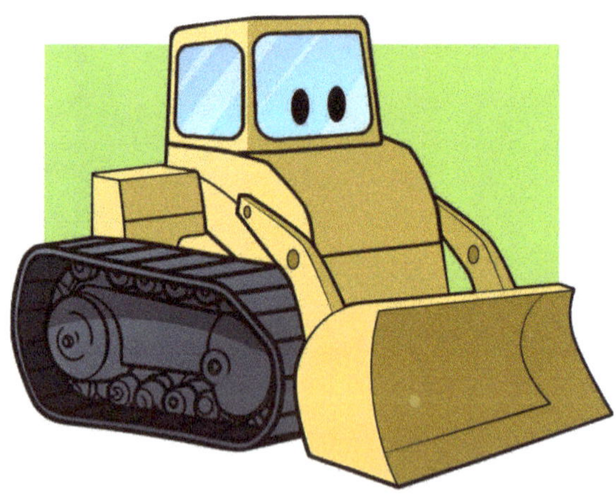

Bring out your best equipment to rebuild!

Something that you will not immediately realize is how tired and totally fatigued you will be due to the chemotherapy which you are using to try to beat your cancer.

This, I call the $100 Bill Factor.

Here is how I explain it. It's like walking across your dining room, seeing a bright, crisp $100 Bill on the floor, and saying to yourself, "Boy, I'd surely like to pick that up sometime."

But you cannot.

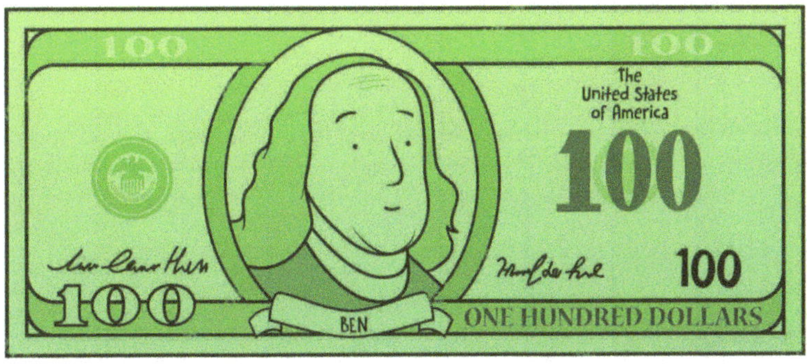

Your body won't let you.

THIS is the FATIGUE you'll experience from all the treatments that you have taken.

My best advice is to jump right on the job of building up your general health from day one.

47

Do everything you can to give your body what it needs to be healthy in every other way. As I've said, take that duty seriously.

It's so easy to just lay around and feel sorry for yourself. For a long time, that is what I did. It was extremely hard to even get up in the morning. I would not even dress in my day clothes when I got up. It just seemed hopeless.

It took a while, but finally, I made the decision that I needed to get my life back. I got up and showered. I shaved. I put skin bracer and underarm lotion on. I dressed in a white shirt, a nice sweater, clean pants, and said to myself, "Get a grip!"

And I did.

I am at my computer right now!

Small accomplishments add up. They keep me going.

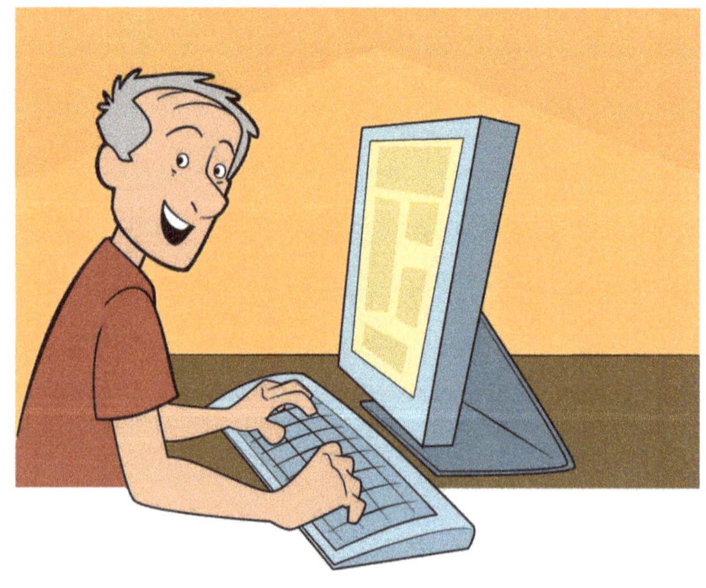

OUR choices. Choices to fix things. To make our bodies healthier.

Fixing what WE put into our bodies; and, what the environment around us put into us that we let stay there.

ONLY GOOD THINGS IN ALL BAD THINGS OUT

My friend keeps telling me, when one is this compromised, this rule cannot be broken – not while one is recovering. Don't consider this a suggestion – it's THAT important.

Repairing years of damage to our bodies due to abuse and neglect is OUR job – not the doctor's.

We've already spoken about one reason why our body is operating in a serious deficit. Improper fuel. Remember, God intended living bodies to self-heal.

I CAN'T GET OVER THAT. ACTUALLY SELF-HEAL! SO MIRACULOUS!

What we eat has always been up to us. Okay, not when Mom was in charge – but I'll bet she made better choices than we've been making.

Unfortunately, often what we eat, even unknown to us, carries bad elements in with it. We haven't really mentioned the bad stuff yet. You probably left those things in because you didn't know how important it was to get rid of them. I know I didn't.

All these chemicals, toxins of all kinds, man-made, processed substances, dyes, etc. are foreign material to your cells. What are they supposed to do with those items? That foreign material interferes with the proper operation of the body.

Our bodies were made to be fed by specific, natural components. When something else is substituted in place of the right, crucial material, we have just sabotaged our marvelous self-healing temple.

No one did it to us. We make conscious choices every day about what goes in and whether to take out anything harmful.

I'm only giving a brief mention, but not going into detail, about things that can cause or contribute to cancer, or of what specific items or practices may remove them, because I'm not a doctor, nutritionist, or a medical practitioner of any medical art.

I'm just trying to give a heads up that, over the ages, exhaustive research has been conducted, and exists, about numerous things which DO contribute to and effect the state of your cancer; and, some methods of their removal, or ways to avoid them.

I AM ONLY NOW BEGINNING TO LEARN how to help myself.

But, if we're going to do this, let's don't go half way.

Buy the premium fuel – not the "knock-off" made with inferior products. Consider avoiding those foods produced with the toxic contaminants in genetically modified foods, glyphosate (like is in Round-Up), pesticides and herbicides.

Let's try to clear out of our bodies all funguses, viruses, Retro-RNA animal viruses, and parasites (bloodworms, round worms, hookworms, tapeworms, threadworms, whipworms, amoebas, protozoa, giardia, salmonella toxoplasmosis, trichinosis, blood flukes, liver flukes, fish flukes, intestinal flukes, and lung flukes).

Parasites are a biggie; there is a LOT of literature supporting the idea that they can play a huge role in cancer. If we are around animals (cats, dogs, horses . . .) or eat food raised with manure, we likely have parasites. Just maybe, they should come out.

This is not an exhaustive list. Many other things can contribute to disease. But, you get the idea. A lot of these burden the body – how badly is dependent on how much, and how often we're exposed to them.

I want you to have hope, like I do, that God has remedies.

When one thinks of remedies, prevention is sometimes over-looked. Just avoid this junk as much as you can. Raise your own food, if possible – or purchase it, hopefully from a trustworthy source – as organically grown as you are able to get.

Buy your supplements from companies who do not get their ingredients from countries known to slide heavy metal contaminants into them.

Keep your home – YOUR SANCTUARY – free from known cancer-contributing offenders. Remove mold, electromagnetic frequencies and radiation.

Read a lot. Study about things that remove heavy metals and parasites. The right food products and herbs do a super job. You'll be amazed about how many help in this task. Read about different formulas and therapies that have helped thousands.

Many people are horribly deficient in the necessary minerals, vitamins, and amino acids. Maybe see what recommended mini-mums are, and if you are meeting those.

Follow health seminars (most are free) online. As they say, knowledge is power.

I've read that infrared saunas are one of the few things which actually CAN remove glyphosate! Check that claim out to see what you find. How wonderful for your body if that works for you. NOTE: A side-effect of those saunas – that even mainstream medical doctors will admit to – is that they can bring high blood pressure numbers down. I LIKE those kind of side-effects! I also read that they help battle cancer.

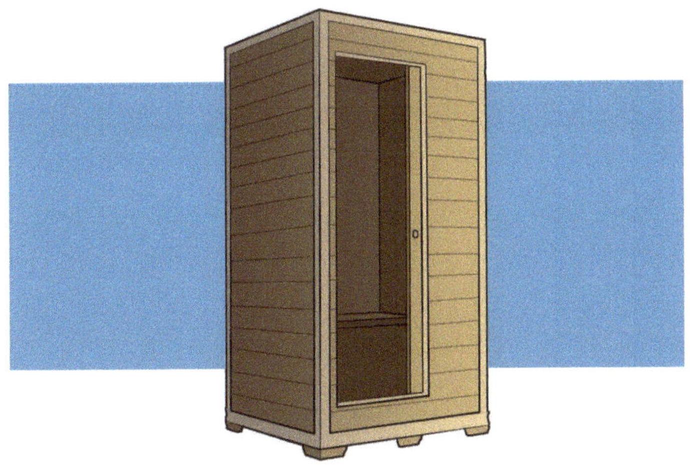

Saunas are not a tool only for the rich. I've heard that the "Y's" sometimes have them. There is a lady locally who charges $3.00 per visit. Check out spas and exercise places. Look around. You'll probably be surprised how available they are.

There are physicians who study and practice ways to clean up the body and restore health. If you are interested in professional help – SEEK THEM OUT.

Just don't feel cancer is hopeless.

This is up to US. Figure out what needs to come out and find ways to accomplish that. There are physicians who specialize in that, books galore on the subject, and frequent, free, online seminars.

Don't be intimidated. This is definitely a job worth doing!

MY FAITH

As I've stated earlier, I did not know how sick I was. When one realizes that fact, it's amazing how quickly one calls on God.

From college days and on for a period of time, one usually does not take their faith as seriously as they should.

I was lucky that I did and am proud to have been an active member of my church. I served the duty of usher in my church for over forty-two years.

Everyone is going to die some time, and when you are told that "You have cancer," you survey the world very differently. I am so thankful that I always had God to count on. This continues to get me through this traumatic time.

I think I realized this most just recently. My neighbor, who is a brain cancer doctor at Ohio State, told my priest just a few weeks ago, "Father, you are looking at a walking miracle."

That surely puts things in perspective as to how very lucky I have been.

I know handling the condition of cancer in your body is difficult and can even feel desolate. I've experienced the ups and downs as things get better and worse.

I also know, not just believe it to be so – but KNOW – how one approaches a situation can make a tremendous difference. Attitude. Confidence that you will make good choices. Boldness on your chosen path. Defiance to all that would defeat you. Do all things with the faith that God is guiding you.

There will be pitfalls. I'm not saying this is easy. I've had my share of bad days. Some really bad days.

Just the word 'cancer' causes fear. It is very important that you do your best to manage it, to try to keep fear out of your mind. When you live in the state of fear, your body is in the sympathetic state. That is the 'fight or flight' response and it shuts down our ability to digest, absorb nutrients, heal and regenerate. This is self-defeating. God can empower you to get past the fear. Let Him.

Absolutely recognize the gravity, but make a positive attitude a priority – only to be topped by faith in God.

While scientific research has been, and still is being done, to study the mind/body connection, no one truly understands how it all works. But work it does. The body influences the mind, and the mind – and emotion – influences the body.

Amazingly, falling in love is a tremendous healer, giving love, accepting love. Generosity. Forgiveness. Peace. Purpose. Gratitude. Meditation in prayer. Doing for others. All healers.

All things God asks us to do every day anyway. Coincidence? I think not. After all, Who most wants His creation to do well!

Don't limit yourself to preconceived notions of how to rid your body of cancer, or of how to help your body tolerate the treatments of radiation and chemo.

Don't stick merely to ideas imposed upon you. Scale the walls to search for ways to support your doctor by nourishing your body between treatments.

We really only have an inkling of the myriad ways God designed our bodies to repair what's wrong. If we only knew what was possible!

Time on earth is a journey. I hope all of our journeys end well.

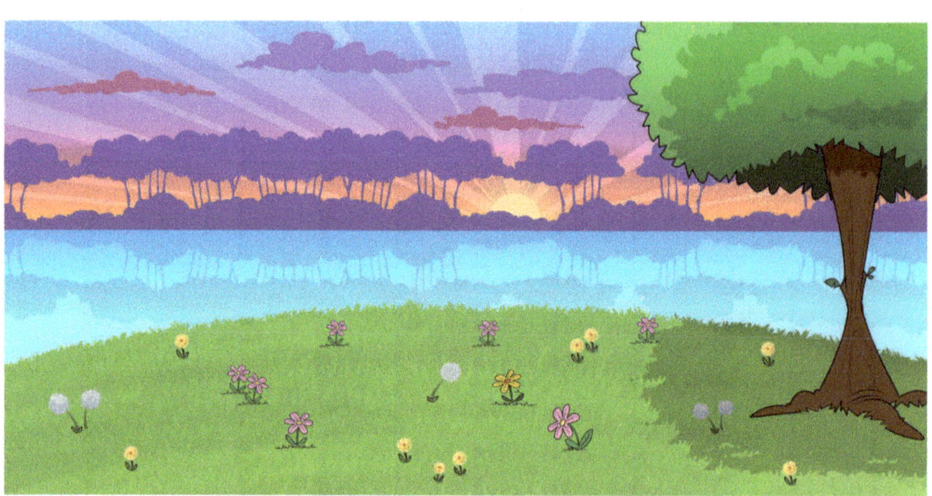

GRATITUDE

I believe gratitude is paramount for peace and healing.

This last chapter is for me.

Perhaps, each of you would like to write your own chapters and surround yourselves with the love you feel for each person in it. Living in love is healing in itself!

I choose to wear my list as a mantle of love.

I have gratitude for:

Robert Paxton, revered father;

Marcella (Fox) Paxton, angelic, patient mother, and, next to God, the most perfect example of love that I know;

Sandy (Buckey) Paxton, she was my wife, possessing amazing intellect, with whom two incredible children were shared; along with twelve grandchildren

CHILDREN AND FAMILIES:
Brett Paxton, wife Leslie and my grandchildren Andrew, George, Charlie and Eliza Paxton

Jennifer (Paxton) Smith, husband Ben, and my grandchildren Ashley, Riley, Matthew, Mary, Bryan, Patrick, Lily and Henry

BROTHERS, SISTERS, THEIR SPOUSES, NIECES AND NEPHEWS:

Anne (Paxton) Owen

Danny and Sandi Paxton and Danny Jr., Melissa and Jessica

John and Lisa Paxton and Dale, Kyle, Bryan, Sean, Colby and Christopher

Joe Paxton

Joan Paxton and husband Alan Kiene and Katy and Alex

I was very fortunate for all the years of love from my family. It was just amazing. I had my dad and mom, that I did not realize as a child, but, looking back, were the blessing of my life.

SPECIAL PERSON:

Lisa Pickett – law paralegal for twenty-eight years and best friend, and, family Bobby, Taylor, Lauren and Cameron, who, too, has helped me with household issues and would help me at a moment's notice

COACHES:

I am so proud to have had three GREAT coaches!

Frank Zubovich, my track coach at Ohio State

Mr. Sam Bates – my high school football coach at Caldwell High School

Mr. Robert Springer – also my high school football coach at Caldwell High School

THE WEXNER MEDICAL CENTER:

I am also grateful to:

Dr. David Bond – my oncologist at OSU, very great doctor, very compassionate and caring – has kept me alive for the past two years

Nurse Leslie and all staff who have been very caring and compassionate

Katie Kiene - administrator at the James who helped me with all appointments and would meet me at the front door entrance to help me to the infusion room

CONCLUDING THOUGHT

I have one hundred people, whom I could call at three in the morning, and they would come.

The commitment that I have had over the years from my associates, college buddies, home town friends, fellow athletic enthusiasts, frat brothers, and so many other close friends, warms my heart.

They have kept me going when times were tough, they have been my constant source of laughter and love.

Words cannot describe how grateful I am for all of you.

Love, Bob

PERSONAL POSTSCRIPT

I had not dealt with cancer as Bob has, so I wanted to explain from where my traditional and alternative health concepts came that I was able to weave around the events in Bob's life.

Bob was familiar and comfortable with the allopathic treatments routinely taught in American Universities, but I had not had total success with the mainstream practice of medicine. Because of our contrasting experiences, this book has an unusual team resulting in viewing wellbeing with divergent lenses.

I've had my own nemesis and for almost thirty years I have researched and experimented on myself to try to get the upper hand over Lyme Disease. Even yet, once in a while, the wee beasties of Lyme, or possibly common co-infections, rear their tenacious heads and cause me trouble.

In 1994-95, when I sought help from our (then) family doctor for a near-debilitating set of ailments, he was unable to find the cause. When he finally decided it was all in my head and wanted to treat me with psychotropic drugs, I told him I was not crazy, I was exhausted, and I began the job of trying to treat myself.

I read and studied every condition I could find that had symptoms similar to mine, trying different formulas, protocols and products. It took several months but, finally, my health returned to near-normal. I have admitted many times that this illness was undoubtedly a blessing to me because of what I learned about wellness and remedies, for both myself and my family.

It was many years before a blood test confirmed Lyme Disease. I spent countless hours reading books and medical articles and devouring data from online seminars which featured doctors and researchers from around the world, addressing both Lyme and cancer. I found the paths of most disorders crossed when one was seeking a return to health instead of just disease management.

When given that frightening cancer diagnosis, one might first take the time to thoughtfully consider if those treatments which cripple the immune system should really be an automatic selection. Perhaps another option might be to at least explore one or more of the numerous therapies and those clinics which offer hopefulness, optimism, and treatment plans to build up and strengthen the body. There is so much more to tell. So much to learn. So many paths of healing.

Even if, after investigating other approaches, the sanctioned methods of conventional medicine become the subsequent choice, the researcher will have gained knowledge of various ways to heal that can become adjunct therapies. That is a good thing.

Consider my part of what was written in this book a brief introduction to only a fragment of what I have encountered in my decades-long adventure. May it plant seeds of curiosity and hope, in all who read this, of what the potential might be in those previously unimagined possibilities.

– Rebecca